Read a Bit! Talk a Bit! Car

Written by Gunilla Denton Cook

Published by Denton Cook Pty Ltd
Copyright Denton Cook Pty Ltd 2013
ABN 5403936874
Sydney Australia
Phone +61 2 9651 3558
Fax   +61 2 9651 3007
Email: dentoncook@bigpond.com
Cover photo by Andrew Cook

Read a Bit! Talk a Bit! is a series of reading activity books intended for people with dementia and/or Alzheimer's disease. The books start with a short article for the group to read, followed by a number of questions for the group leader to ask and engage the participants in conversation to encourage personal and meaningful reminiscences to flow.

All the reading pages are in large type, 44 pt, and the text is only on one page per spread in order to help the individual to concentrate on the text and to minimise the constraints of visual impairment.

Memories recalled from earlier in life are often very therapeutic for all and especially for people with memory impairment. These questions are formulated to create meaningful engagement with the past. Remembering increases self esteem and a feeling of positive worth as the participants recall personal experiences.

This series of books successfully achieve this thanks to the range of familiar topics and questions to prompt and encourage discussions.

Titles available:

At the Movies	Lawnmower	Scissors
Cake	Money	Soup
Cat	Pencil	Stamps
Chickens	Perfume	Teddy Bear
Dog	Safety Pin	Telephone
Garden	Sandwich	

To have your own car means freedom, for most of us. It opens so many opportunities to come and go when we please. It may be for work, or just to go for a picnic, because the mood takes us.

Pass to next reader

When the first successful gasoline engine was created, cars were soon seen as a 'must have' among the upper classes.

Pass to next reader

The production of cars started in the late eighteen hundreds. Thirty American car manufacturers produced two thousand and five hundred cars between them, in 1899.

Pass to next reader

A few years later, in 1908, Henry Ford released his Model T.

Business was booming for Mr Ford and his creation.

He was quoted in the press: 'I will build a motorcar for the great multitude.' And so he did.

Pass to next reader

He improved the speed of the assembly line for the chassis from over twelve hours down to an hour and a half. Ford produced more cars than any other company at the time. Between the years 1909 and 1927 the Ford Motor Company built more than fifteen million cars.

__Pass to next reader__

During World War II, most car manufacturers around the world worked for the armed forces and not many civilian cars were produced.

Pass to next reader

In the fifties, the American cars were large and often referred to as gas-guzzlers. The biggest sellers in the USA during the fifties were Chevrolet, closely followed by Ford.

**Pass to next reader**

Read a Bit! Talk a Bit! Dog written by Gunilla Denton Cook.
©2013 Denton Cook Pty Ltd

In Europe, the cars were smaller. One of the biggest sellers was the small car, Morris Minor. There are many of these cars still on the roads today, driven by enthusiasts of the original model.

Pass to next reader

The next model of the Morris Minor was the Mini. This was a very successful car. It is small, but it has a lot of power. It was used and loved by all, including rally drivers. The Mini won the Monte Carlo Rally four times.

Pass to next reader

Cars today are far more advanced than Ford's first Model T was. Our vehicles today have GPS, rear view cameras, heated seats and many more conveniences and technical advantages. The car has come a long way in the past one hundred years.

__Pass to group leader__

Questions

1. How old were you the first time you travelled in a car?

2. If your parents had a car, what kind was it?

3. What colour was it?

4. Was it your mother or your father who mainly drove the car?

5. How many cars did you have in your family?

6. How old were you when you got your driver's licence?

7. What make and colour was your first car?

8. Did you buy a new car or a used one?

9. What kind of car is your favourite?

10. How many cars have you had?

11. Have you ever had a car accident? If so, was anyone hurt?

12. How much did a tank full of petrol cost for your first car?

13. How far was the longest trip you have travelled by car?

14. When and where did you get your driver's licence?

15. Do you prefer a manual or an automatic gearbox? Why?

16. Did you have any funny or frightening experiences teaching someone to drive?

17. Who taught you to drive?

18. How many fines have you had for traffic offenses?

19.   What do you always make sure you have in the car?

(Water, umbrella, etc.)

20.   Can you name a car for every letter of the alphabet?

A   Alfa Romeo, Aston Martin, Audi
B   BMW, Bentley, Bugatti, Buick
C   Cadillac, Chevrolet, Chrysler, Corvette, Capri
D   Daimler, Dodge, Datsun
E   Eagle
F   Ford, Fiat, Ferrari
G   GMC, GEO
H   Honda, Hummer, Hyundai, Holden
I   Isuzu
J   Jaguar, Jeep
K   Kia
L   Lincoln, Lexus, Lamborghini, Land Rover
M   Mercedes, Mazda, Mini, Morris Minor,
N   Nissan
O   Opel, Oldsmobile
P   Porsche, Plymouth, Pontiac
Q
R   Rolls Royce, Rover, Range Rover
S   Subaru, Saab, Seat, Skoda, Suzuki
T   Toyota, Triumph, Tesla
U
V   Volkswagen, Volvo, Vauxhall
W   Wanderer, Wolseley
X
Y   Yamaha
Z   Zephyr

www.ingramcontent.com/pod-product-compliance
Lightning Source LLC
Chambersburg PA
CBHW081813280526
45789CB00008B/3111